DEDICATION

To all my beautiful readers

Disclaimer

DRINK smoothie! HAVE A NICE DAY

Contents

INTRODUCTION

BENEFITS OF A SMOOTHIE LIFESTYLE

There are numerous benefits of the smoothies. They are extremely healthy and really easy to make, and they can change your life in many ways.

Leading a healthy life involves many things. If you want to be successful on the daily basis and feel prepared and energized to do the activities, and if you want to enjoy doing things during the day, your body needs regular exercise and above all healthy diet. There are many ways to keep your body in good shape. You can go to the gym, also go jogging, doing yoga or tai chi, or something similar. You just have to find out what suits you the most.

Practicing is definitely important if you want to lead a healthy life but if you really want to change something healthy diet is a very important element, maybe even crucial. In order to have healthy and balanced diet you should know how to properly practice different nutrients. This considers the right amount of healthy fatty acids, vitamins, carbohydrates, proteins, etc.

In order to accomplish this you should add smoothies into your daily diet. They are like a true health bomb for your organism. Smoothies will keep your organism hydrated, give you power and energy, they are perfect for your skin, digestion and many other things. Consume them and you'll enjoy many health benefits. I believe you will find everything you need in smoothies. For example you can lose weight in a healthy and natural way, your skin will look better, I may freely say great.

Smoothies are not expensive. If you are worried about preparation, it's actually easy to make them. You get to choose the ones you like because there is a whole bunch of different combinations. By consuming them you'll have the long lasting energy. Include them into your day as a meal replacement or a snack and you won't have to worry about not getting enough vitamins, minerals, magnesium, proteins, everything you need. For those who are not kitchen fans they will be great because they are easily and fast prepared. One of the advantages is that it won't matter which season it is, you can make them out of frozen ingredients but if possible choose fresh, depending on where you are and what part of the year it is. And, best of all, your kids will love them.

WHY DAIRY-FREE SMOOTHIES

There are a many smoothie recipes (which are easily available) that are based on the usage of different types of protein powders (because they are rich in proteins) or yogurt, but if you are a type of person who wants to live a life that is dairy-free this just won't work. We will all agree that proteins are an important nutrient, especially of great value for healing, repair, growth and many other things. Dairy products are a great source of proteins indeed, but if you want dairy-free diet you don't have to be scared, there is a way of providing necessary daily intake of proteins.

Fabulous is the fact that there and vegan products you can use as a substitute in your smoothies. Some of them are hemp seeds, coconut yogurt, chia seeds, many protein powders, nuts, beans (believe it or not) and even some vegetables can give you enough proteins. So, dairy-based food is not obligatory.

Once we decide to change our lifestyle, especially when we think about changing some eating habits, we first think whether we'll have everything we need (vitamins, minerals, proteins, etc.). If we talk about dairy-free products, first thing we are worried about is "Will I get enough proteins?". Well, of course you will. As previously mentioned there are numerous nutrients and products that are not dairy-based but will still give you all the proteins you need.

In case you are wondering why dairy-free smoothies I can tell you that there are many reasons why exactly should we use dairy-free smoothies. Some people need to switch their diet because of the intolerance on the dairy-based products (glucose). On the other hand, other people have different reasons such as: they don't like them, or they have problems with digestion and can't stand the dairy-based products and many other reasons. One of them might be clean skin, too. If you want to help your skin repair and make it look like baby's skin, delete, or at least avoid dairy-based products. It's not necessary to use milk or yogurt to make a good and tasty smoothie.

Independent on the reasons you have to, or you want to avoid or exclude dairy-based nutrients, be aware of the fact that there are many nutrients similar to them that are natural source of proteins you need during the day.

SMOOTHIES AS MEAL REPLACEMENT OR JUST A SNACK?

Frequently asked question among people who want to change their eating habits is whether a smoothie should replace our meal or not. The important thing with preparing smoothies is that we use the whole vegetable or fruit. That is one of the best things when it comes to smoothies because this way we combine all the ingredients together. Food prepared like this is full of fibers which can keep you satiated long period of time. You can also combine it with some other stuff such as butter (peanut) or avocado. Not only these, but many other ingredients are great and will keep you satiated. Smoothies can also be combined with different types of fruit.

The reason I can tell you that smoothies can be a meal replacement is because they can provide your organism everything it needs. They contain healthy ingredients and above all everything you should have in one meal. They will give you enough energy, enough power, etc.

But, of course, it's not necessary to replace your meals with smoothies. If you are not interested in replacing a meal with a smoothie, then just don't. Have it as a snack. It will equally good for your organism. The important thing is to add them to your daily diet, one way or another. Have them before breakfast. Have them instead of your dinner or try them as your snack. It really doesn't matter, just take them.

If your choice is to use the smoothies as an actual meal, the breakfast time is the best time to do this. It will give you all the necessary ingredients that will provide you with enough energy and calories up until lunch time.

If you don't want to substitute breakfast for a smoothie than take it while out or at work instead of some fast food full of carbohydrates lunch which is, as we all know, the unhealthiest thing you can eat.

If we talk about dinner you may try to avoid drinking smoothies in this part of the day. You can do this sometimes but if you are already trying to change something than choose breakfast or lunch time as the best solution.

My advice is to include smoothies in your daily routine. As a meal or a snack, all the same, the important is to consume something healthy and smoothies are a great start. Bon appétit.

WHAT NOT TO ADD TO YOUR SMOOTHIES

People sometimes think that everything healthy can and should be mixed together. Unfortunately, that's not the case. There are and many different rules of how to combine ingredients. This is very important when it comes to smoothies. Why? Well, as I've already mentioned there are certain rules of how to combine the ingredients. Some of the ingredients are simple not for use in blenders or juicer. Some of them might spoil the taste. So, be careful. It doesn't mean that if something is good for you and your organism must be a part of your smoothie. I'll give you a short list of things that you shouldn't put in your smoothies.

Don't mix cilantro and kale. Don't add mustard greens to your smoothie. Yes, they are full of nutrition but if they are not cooked, they've really got a specific spicy taste that not even the sweetest fruit can mask it. Use kale or baby spinach when making your green smoothie. My advice is to save them for stir-fries instead.

Ginger, the fresh one, is one more ingredient you should avoid adding to your smoothie. If you really want to add it, make sure to finely mince or grate it and then add it.

Then celery. It might taste great to nibble it but it will be really yucky when you add it to your smoothie and drink it. Trust me!

One more foodstuff to avoid here is raw beets. Yes, I know, it's pretty and attractive but never the less. If you really want to add it, make sure to cook and peel it first.

If you want whole dates, my answer is no. Chop them first and then soak them for 15 to 20 minutes to soften them up first.

The next thing to avoid would be ice. Yeah, you've heard me, ice. Some of you believe that a smoothie needs ice but that just not true. Actually, the drink is better off without it. The ice will dilute your smoothie and make it watery. It can also damage the blades of your blender. If you want a cold smoothie take frozen fruit or some cold liquids.

Sugar, especially white, is bad for our organism in many ways. It's the worst ingredient you can use when making smoothies. You should avoid all types of juices, even if they are totally made of fruit. They can only stop you from losing weight. If you are using some kind of powders such as for example protein ones, make sure (check twice) that there is no refined sugar or any other sugars like evaporated cane juice, syrup, brown rice syrup, etc. Some of them are not so bad but they've got many calories and because of that will raise up your blood sugar and hinder you weight loss.

Fruit is known as a healthy food but you put too much of it into your smoothie (more than one cup is too much) you definitely take too much sugar (I know it's natural, but you should be careful with it as well). Calories found in sugar aren't efficient in building muscles and burning fat like those found in proteins, fibers or healthy fats. So, avoid more than a cup per smoothie and if possible choose the ones low in sugar such as berries. If you want to sweeten your smoothie, try liquid stevia- less refined and calorie-free).

You like nut butters? Especially peanut butter? I understand, I really do! I love it. But, there are so many nut butters out there; maybe you could try something different. Nuts are great source of proteins and healthy fats, so don't be afraid to include them in your diet for more benefits. Instead of peanut butter, you can try almond as a great alternative. It's great.

Be careful when choosing yogurt. Fat-free and unsweetened yogurt is ok to add into your smoothie, like almond based, coconut or organic soy yogurt. If it's from a dairy source make sure it's nonfat and without sugar.

Many people add protein powders to their smoothies, so do I. But there are some things you should pay attention to if using them. Choose organic and raw forms of powders without sweeteners, soy, dairy, additives. You don't need them in your smoothies.

When it comes to carbs, they aren't something you should completely avoid. If you want to add them, chose those whose carb content comes from fibers not sugar. You can use hemp seeds, chia seeds, leafy greens, low sugar fruit, etc.

If you like milk but your goal is losing weight, use nondairy milk. It's high in calories and sugar. If it's possible, make your own almond or coconut milk.

There are more things you should avoid when making smoothies, that's for sure. I chose some of them to bring you into the world of a healthy life.

SOAKING YOUR NUTS, SEEDS AND OATS

You probably wonder why soaking nuts, seeds and outs in some recipes. The process of soaking at home means imitating nature's germination of a seed into a plant. At first it seems odd doing this. But there are many reasons for this and let's see them.

Soaking nuts, seed, grains helps increase the activity of phytic acid which is found in grains and nuts. This acid inhibits nutrient and mineral absorption in the body. It's not unusual that in plant-based diet we have lacking of some very important things such as calcium, minerals, vitamins (especially B), iron, zinc and others.

Soaking is very popular in row food diets, as well as vegetarian and vegan diets. There is a good reason why. Any process that can increase the nutrient content (no matter how small it is) in a restricted diet is a great idea. By restricted, I'm referring to restriction of certain food groups that normally contain heaps of these precious minerals like iron, calcium, zinc, and other.

Nuts, seeds, and grains are full of nutrients. But in order to protect ourselves from natural toxins that exist in them for their protection but harm us, they need to be soaked and dehydrated. This is extremely beneficial to our health. It removes anti-nutrients from them such as tannin, goitrogens, then phytates. It helps neutralization of inhibitor enzymes. It also increases the power of some nutrients (B vitamin) and makes proteins more available. It removes toxins and helps the growth of some beneficial bacteria essential for our health. Then, it promotes the growth of healthy enzymes vital for healthy digestion.

Nuts, seeds, grains are one of the greatest gifts we've got. They naturally protect themselves. To ensure their own survival, nuts, grains and seeds contain some inner toxic inhibitors that protect the plant from germination. But once they get wet and there is sufficient moisture that they germinate.

This is a natural protective phenomenon. It is a wonderful thing for the survival of the foods. But it's highly necessary to neutralize these protective toxins before consumption. This is very important for our digestive system. Have you noticed how after eating a lot of nuts or seeds you've got a horrible stomach ache?

There are many more reasons why soaking is great. Doing this with raw nuts and seeds increases the nutritional content of vitamins (A, C and specially vitamin B). Soaking nuts or seeds in warm water (salted a bit) activates the enzymes that neutralize the inhibitors making them easier to digest.

If you want to save nuts and seeds for later you need to dehydrate or dry them. If you want to use them in smoothies you can just soak and rinse. I do that all the time. If you are preparing milk for smoothies just soak, rinse, blend and eat.

Here is an advice that might encourage you to soak: soaking whole grains actually really softens them up and makes them fluffier. This can make a huge difference in taste. Try, you might be pleasantly surprised.

When you chose your nuts, seeds, oats, please, make sure they are organic.

How to soak?

Put the nuts or seeds in a glass bowl and cover them with warm, filtered water with a teaspoon of sea salt absorbed in it (2:1- 2 parts water to 1 part nuts or seeds).Keep the bowl covered with some thin cloth at room temperature recommended period of time. All toxic enzyme inhibitors will stay in soaking water.

TIPS ON FREEZING YOUR FRUITS

Maybe you've thought that you can just throw fruits in a freezer bag and your job is done. Well, no. If you do this, fruit often freezes together into one brick. The first problem comes when you need just a few cups to make a dessert or want to use them in your tasty smoothie. Thawing the fruit like this turns them into a watery mess.

Much better and easier way to freeze fresh fruits is to first prepare them just as you would if you were going to use them immediately. If you are freezing apples and pears peel and core them first. If you want to freeze peaches, remove the pits and chop them into small pieces (in size of a bite). Berries and other small fruits leave whole. Then freeze all the fruits on a baking sheet in a single layer.

It may look tough but it's actually very easy. Just follow few steps when freezing the fruit and you will have your precious nutrients even if their season is far away. This way you will preserve not only look but the taste too. So, let's repeat.

Thoroughly wash and dry fruit

If the fruit has a skin, peel it. Remove all the undesirable spots

If your fruit is big (peaches), cut or slice it into smaller pieces (your choice)

Remove as much moisture as possible (use a towel)

Spread fruit into a single layer

Cover with plastic cling wrap, move to the freezer for several hours

Remove your tray from freezer

Peel the fruit off the paper (gently), and transfer to labeled freezer bags. Squeeze as much air as possible out of freezer bags before. And now your fruit is ready to go, and it will last for 6 to 9 months.

There are few things to remember about certain fruits. Sweet apples tend to hold their flavor better in the freezer than tart ones. Peel and slice them before freezing. If you want to freeze a large batch then soak the apples into salty water. If you want to freeze berries (blackberries, blueberries, raspberries, strawberries), wash them first then dry thoroughly before freezing and always freeze them whole. Bananas should be peeled first then sliced. You should do the same with kiwi, mangoes, pineapple and peaches. You don't have to peel apricots. Cherries should be pitted before freezing.

The best method for saving lemons, oranges or grapefruit is to save the skin and juice separately.

BUILDING THE SMOOTHIE HABIT

The hardest part after bringing the decision to lead a healthier life is where to start. It's not easy to change habits, especially when it comes to food. Drinking smoothies can be an easy and enjoyable way to increase the intake of vegetables, fruits, and other healthy foods. I'll give you few tips that can make your blending easier whether you are new in making smoothies, or have been drinking them for years. When something is easy it's not hard to accept it. These tips can make preparing smoothies easier and faster. Considering the fact we are all different and want different things, choose what the easiest way for you is.

First, **keep your recipes simple.** You don't have to add everything to every smoothie. You can focus on certain flavors that can improve the taste. If you use fewer ingredients you will speed up preparation time. Instead of putting everything in every smoothie, make different combinations. This way you can see what your favorite taste is, what you like and what you don't like.

Second, prepare your smoothie ahead. This will save your time, and can especially be useful if you have to rush to get out of the house in the morning. There are a few different ways to do this. You can blend a bigger batch and keep it in the fridge. Off course it's better to take it fresh, but if there's not enough time, any smoothie is better than no smoothie. **You can also** put all the ingredients (except for liquid and frozen) in blender the night before, and store it in a fridge. You can freeze the ingredients as well; just don't add any liquids until the preparation time.

Make sure your blender is always accessible. This may sound funny but the fact is that it is easier when it's close to us and available.

Just like blender, keep smoothie ingredients on hand so you're always ready to blend!

If you get bored with your smoothies, look for new ways to spice up your blends. Find new recipes, remove one or add one ingredient. Even if it's just one, it may bring a new life to your smoothie.

If you are building a smoothie habit you have to be aware that this is not something you will do for a month or two. This is something it should become a part of your life, routine (like brushing teeth). Once you accept this as a part of your life, things will be much easier.

ON SUPERFOODS, SEEDS AND POWDERS

Many discussions about superfoods have been led during the past few years especially about seeds.

Let's see about chia seeds! They are but are incredibly healthy. They contain fibers and proteins. You can use them to prepare chia see smoothies. Chia seeds are also a great source of calcium and Omega-3 fatty acids. They contain more calcium than milk, more iron than spinach, more magnesium than broccoli. Use them in your smoothies, you won't regret.

Pumpkin seeds contain almost half the recommended dose of magnesium in just one quarter of ¼ a cup. They are also a rich in zinc that. Zink is vital for skin, cell growth, and immunity. When you are making a smoothie, throw a handful of pumpkin seeds in and enjoy.

Sunflower seeds are a great source of B Vitamins including. They can help you promote immune system. They are also a source of Vitamin E (important for healthy skin). They are also good because of copper, selenium and magnesium. It's my friendly advice to include them into your everyday diet.

There is a variety of superfood powders accessible today. Make sure when choosing and buying them, double-check that they are of organic origin. They can be great since they are rich nutrients, antioxidants, anti-carcinogens, vitamins and minerals.

They can be a great addition to your smoothie. There is really a great variety of these powders available. Be careful when choosing and enjoy preparing healthy smoothies.

SMOOTHIES FOR HEALTH CONDITIONS

Smoothies are superfoods! They are nutritional powerhouses that deserve are a special place in your daily diet. They are packed with nutrients and able to improve your health in so many ways.

I could write you all day about the benefits of all the ingredients you could mix in your smoothie but here I will give you just a short introduction. I believe this will give you enough reasons to start introducing them into your daily diet. Superfood smoothies will make you feel great and look better than ever. Every one of them will give you something good.

Berries are the fruits that are great natural antioxidants. Any type, blueberries, blackberries, acai, and others are super. I would highly recommend acai (if available to you). These dark red fruits contain more antioxidants than any other food we know (such as dark chocolate, red wine, blueberries, etc.). It has few calories, a lot of, proteins, minerals, fiber. They help in lowering cholesterol, preventing atherosclerosis, and even killing cancer cells. You can use the frozen pulp of acai in your smoothies without adding other ingredients or mix it with other fruits or cacao.

For lowering cholesterol, slowing tumor growth, preventing kidney stones, improving digestion, relieving constipation, stabilizing blood sugar levels try aloe vera. For your smoothies you can use aloe vera. Cut back the outside of the leaves to get to the gel inside. You can add it to any smoothie without changing the taste.

Cacao increases blood flow, lower bad cholesterol levels raising levels of the good one, , regulate blood sugar, lower blood pressure and improves brain function, and mood (that's why chocolate is so good). Do not hesitate to add cacao to your smoothie, but remember it won't be sweet. Raw cacao is bitter and you'll need to add a little natural sweetener.

Chia seeds are a great source of fiber. This makes them perfect for weight loss or weight maintenance. Omega-3 and omega-6 fatty acids are also an important part of chia seeds. They are also high in protein and several important minerals. Just add a couple of tablespoons of them to your smoothies and you will get many benefits. They can as well control your blood sugar levels, prevent blood clots, and reduce high blood pressure. I've told you, so many benefits in just one ingredient.

It's a real surprise how many benefits comes from coconut oil. Coconut oil has been proven to aid weight loss, lower bad cholesterol and even help to reverse the course of Alzheimer's disease. It also has an antibiotic effect. Some studies show that it can help you kill the bacteria that cause acne. You can preserve it longer than other oils. Add a tablespoon to a chocolate or fruit smoothie and enjoy the flavor and benefits of coconut.

Goji berries are high in vitamins, minerals, protein, and antioxidants. They are perfect for vegetarians and vegans. They can help protect you from heart disease and improve your eye health. They can improve your immune system and even help with serious autoimmune disorders. They taste fantastic in all fruit-based smoothies.

Honey is one more ingredient great for your smoothie and beneficial for your health. It contains antioxidants and has strong antibacterial properties. It helps with allergies. It is also a good source of protein, vitamins, and minerals. It is also used to treat asthma, anemia, acne, arthritis and many other diseases. Honey is easily added to smoothies and can be one of your natural sweeteners.

Since I've shown the great impact of smoothies (each one of them) on your organism I encourage you to start exploring the wonderful world of smoothies. Try them; mix them, read different recipes. You will most certainly find the ones good for your problems, tasty and perfect for your organism.

Every ingredient has its own advantages. Some are full of vitamins (A, B, C, E). Many of them have inflammatory power (such as tropical fruit). They can also help your digestive system (pineapple) or improve your immune system. They will also reduce cholesterol, blood pressure or relax your muscles. Grape and parsley will protect your bones and teeth (Can you believe it?) because they are full of vitamin K. They will provide you with energy clean your skin, even reduce the amount of stress. Also, they are essential for a healthy brain. They will lower risk for many diseases, like cancer. Even fresh herbs (mint, basil, rosemary) are great, especially as antioxidants.

All these, and many others can be added to smoothies. The number of variations is endless. Choose what you like, mix them, try a new one every day. Enjoy preparing smoothies and at the same time give your organism everything it needs to resist bad influences.

FAT BURNING WITH SMOOTHIES

This is one very common question and the answer is yes, smoothies can help you in burning fat and losing weight. First, you need to know that this is a long time process. You have to make an effort if you want to see some real and permanent results. You must lose more calories than you take in.

The first thing to know about smoothies is that they are made to be tasty. If you add the fact they are good for you, you won't find better combination. Many of them can be beneficial for your health and at the same time help you burn fat. For this, it is very important to choose what you put in your smoothie. There are some things like yogurt (nondairy) and various other ingredients which are natural fat fighters and will help you eliminate unwanted body fat.

Don't be scared, they aren't yucky. These smoothies are delicious and at the same time easy to make. You can have them for breakfast because they will fill you up with energy and will burn fat. They are also good for a healthy and easily made dessert. There is no better choice if you want to lose weight.

When you're trying to lose weight and burn fat your first choice should be green smoothies. They are nutrient powerhouses. By combining them you can get one tasty drink. Most of green smoothies are low-calorie. Use them as a substitute for unhealthy foods and you can lose weight. The ideal would be to combine green smoothies as a replacement for one or two meals. Combine them with other healthy foods; avoid fats and other high-calorie but low-nutrient food and practice. Accomplishment won't drop behind.

Use spinach, avocado, and more, to provide a healthy dose of ingredients.

Too much fat is not only ugly but also dangerous for our health. It can cause serious different problems such as asthma, cancer, cardiovascular problems, diabetes and many other diseases.

The best way to avoid gaining weight or to lose fat is to accept a healthy lifestyle. Include nutrient-dense smoothies. Let them be a part of your daily routine. Accept at once that nothing happens overnight.

Besides green smoothies there are many others that you can use if you want to lose fat. Try smoothies with berries with a heap of proteins which will help to burn fat. All you have to do is toss the ingredients in your blender and process for just a few seconds.

If you are a fan of green tea, you should know that alone has many good fat burning properties and if you pair it with blueberries, you'll get a double-score. Coconut milk is also a great natural fat fighter.

Now you see there are many smoothies that will help you lose weight and burn fat. You just have to pick up your recipe and get started. It may take a while but if you are determined in changing your lifestyle from unhealthy to healthy you will succeed. Good luck!

SMOOTHIE TO GO!

Streamlining the process makes it even easier, especially if you are really pressed for time in the morning. Prepare whatever you can ahead of time – what I do is to portion out the nuts and seeds that I will be using for the week ahead and store them in little containers. I do the same with the fruit and freeze it ahead of time. Smoothie to Go Streamlining the process makes it even easier, especially if you are really pressed for time in the morning. Prepare whatever you can ahead of time – what I do is to portion out the nuts and seeds that I will be using for the week ahead and store them in little containers. I do the same with the fruit and freeze it ahead of time.

IMPROVE DIGESTION

Now, let's talk about digestion. Digestion is something that all of us do. We're all human, and we eat food, so we have to break it down into tinier particles in order to get the nutrients out of it. Simple, right? You've probably heard that in your health classes back in the day. Well smoothies can actually help with those who have a poor digestion, and it can help improve the health of that. Simply put, many smoothies are already broken down in order to help relieve chewing. That makes it easier on you, and it's already usually crushed into tinier pieces. Once they're brown up, they go down into your stomach, and the nutrients are directly absorbed. This puts less tension on your intestines, and if you get indigestion, you'll be able to relieve that with this. Smoothies can actually help clean the gut out and get rid of the blockage and tension that is present in the intestines. Another benefit that it can have is that it can also clean the gut out through the use of probiotics in the smoothies. You can get fruits that have natural probiotics within, but it can also be done by purchasing probiotics. Probiotics are used to help clean out the gut so that the bad bacteria and toxins move out of the body and are replaced by the good bacteria. You can actually use this to help clean out the toxins in the body by taking it with a smoothie. Simply put, you can mix in the probiotics and blend it with the food. This is actually better for you because it will make taking them in easier, because they ca be a bit strong for most people. Once you have that within you, then you can let it clean out your gut. Plus, with the fruits and vegetables in the body, you're allowing natural foods within there, and it will make your life all the more easier. It's actually miraculous what it can do for you, and you'll be able to have the health benefits that you've always dreamed of. You can improve digestion health with a smoothie, and you can include other fruits and vegetables in order to improve the system and to make digestion all the more better. Doing this can change your life, and it's another major benefit of including smoothies in the diet you have.

RECIPES

Mango-Strawberry Smoothie

Great things really do come in small packages. This creamy mango based smoothie offers tons of health benefits for your whole body.

Prep Time: 10 minutes
Servings: 1

Ingredients:
2 mangoes, cubed and frozen
½ c strawberries, stemmed and frozen
1 tbsp lime juice
1 tsp lime zest, finely grated
1 tbsp honey OR agave syrup
½ c coconut water

Instructions:
Add all ingredients to your blender and blend until smooth. If too thick, add more coconut water. If too thin, add more frozen strawberries.

Rocket Fuel Smoothie

As the name says, this smoothie is pure rocket fuel! Whether you are getting ready to work out, just finishing your workout or getting ready for another busy day, this is a quick and easy power-up packed with all kinds of nutrients.

Prep Time: 5 minutes

Servings: 2

Ingredients:

1 c pomegranate juice

½ c beets, peeled and grated

1 c raspberries, frozen

1 c cherries, pitted and frozen

½ Hass avocado

1 tbsp chia seeds

½ c coconut milk

2 tsp fresh ginger, minced

dash of cayenne pepper

Instructions:

Mix all ingredients together in your blender and process until smooth.

Pink Power Smoothie

Sweet, tangy and earthy, this smoothie is very satisfying and healthy for you. It boosts liver function which will make your skin glow with health and make your digestive system very happy. Besides, it tastes delicious!

Prep Time: 5 minutes
Servings: 2

Ingredients:
1 c unsweetened apple juice
½ c pomegranate juice
½ c beet, peeled and grated
1 c blueberries, frozen
1 banana, sliced and frozen
1 scoop vanilla protein powder

Instructions:
Put all ingredients in your blender and blend on high until smooth. For a creamier smoothie you can add 1 c plain yogurt.

Sweet Zing Orange Smoothie

Filled with detoxifying ingredients and high levels of antioxidants, this smoothie cleans the blood and boosts your immune system to let you function better all day long. Gorgeously orange, sweet to the taste and with a zip of warmth from the ginger, you'll feel wonderfully refreshed as this nutrient packed drink is also excellent at hydrating your cells.

Prep Time: 10 minutes

Servings: 3

Ingredients:

1 c carrot juice

1 orange, peeled, sectioned and frozen

2 bananas, sliced and frozen

1 c pineapple chucks, frozen

½ c fresh spinach, tightly packed

¼ tsp turmeric powder

1 inch piece of fresh ginger, grated

ice cubes, as needed

Instructions:

Place all ingredients into your blender and puree on high until smooth. For a creamier smoothie, add ½ c yogurt or almond milk. Ice cubes only need to be added to thicken the mixture after initial blending.

Tropical Green Smoothie

This sweet-tart smoothie comes with a tropical twist that will have you doing the limbo in no time. Sweet mango and tangy pineapple mingle with mint and lime that will make you forget this smoothie is healthy!

Prep Time: 10 minutes

Servings: 2

Ingredients:

2 c coconut water

1 mango, peeled, pitted, cubed and frozen

1 c pineapple chunks, frozen

2 c fresh spinach, tightly packed

¼ c fresh mint leaves, tightly packed and stems removed

1 tbsp lime juice

10 ice cubes

Instructions:

Add all ingredients to your blender, beginning on low speed work up to high until smooth.

Ginger-Plum Fairy Smoothie

If you are following a diet with a lot of raw vegetables in it, you are probably experiencing fluctuations in your body's temperature regulation. Plums are rich in fiber and other nutrients that are good for your digestion and along with the warmth of ginger and kick of cayenne, this smoothie will help you warm up from the inside out as it boosts your metabolism.

Prep Time: 10 minutes

Servings: 2

Ingredients:

1 c almond milk

2 tbsp hemp seeds

2 tbsp chia seeds

2 tbsp almond butter

1 tbsp coconut butter

¼ tsp pumpkin pie spice

1 tbsp fresh ginger, peeled and grated

1 ½ c plums, cubed and frozen

½ c beet root, peeled and grated raw OR cooked till tender

6 ice cubes

Instructions:

Blend all ingredients except ice cubes for 30 seconds. Add ice and process until smooth and creamy.

Tangy Tropical Fruits

A flavorful and refreshing smoothie that will help keep your body and skin from ageing so fast. It is perfect for hot summer days as a snack or for breakfast.

Nutritional Info: Calories 175, Fat 1.6 g, Protein 6.6 g, Carbs 36.1 g
Servings:2
Prep Time: 15 minutes

Ingredients:
1/2 cup chopped, peeled carrots
1 cup peeled, chopped frozen mango
1 kiwi peeled and chopped
1/2 cup peeled and chopped melon
1/2 cup canned papaya
1/2 papaya juice (use the juice from the papaya can)
1/2 cup green tea
1/2 cup Greek yogurt
1 tablespoon powder cinnamon
6 ice cubes

Directions:
1. Put the ice cubes into the blender and pulse for a few seconds.

2. Add the rest of the ingredients and blend until the smoothie is well blended.

3. Pour into tall glasses and decorate with a slice of lemon.

Fruity Antioxidant Delight

A smoothie with incredible antioxidant power from the berries and awesome digestive benefits from chia seeds. This rich blend makes for a delicious breakfast and will also help to cleanse your stomach of toxins.

Nutritional Info: Calories 272, Fat 5.2g, Protein 8.4 g, Carbs 53.2g

Servings: 2

Prep Time: 10 minutes

Ingredients:
1 cup frozen blackberries
4 cups spinach
1 peach
1 apple
3 plums
1 teaspoon chia seeds
1 cup blueberries
1 cup water
1 cup natural yogurt
4 ice cubes

Directions:
1. Remove the peach's pit and the apple's core.
2. Put the ice cubes into the blender and pulse for a few seconds to break them a little.

3. Add the remaining ingredients into the blender, except for the chia seeds.

4. Blend until the mixture is well combined.

5. Serve in tall glasses and add the chia seeds.

Chocolate And Acai Booster

The ultimate antioxidant smoothie recipe that will change your breakfasts forever. Start your day off with a tall glass of this smoothie, load your body with protein, vitamins, mood boosting chemicals and minerals. Discover why acai and cocoa powder are considered super food.

Nutritional Info: Calories 310, Fat 13.3 g, Protein 7.0 g, Carbs 47.3 g

Servings: 1

Prep Time: 10 minutes

Ingredients:

1 cup strawberries

1 cup frozen cherries

1 tablespoon acai powder

1 tablespoon cocoa powder

1 tablespoon almond butter

1/2 cup rice milk Water (as needed)

4 ice cubes

Directions:

1. Wash the strawberries and remove their leafy heads.

2. Throw all the ingredients into the blender.

3. Blend for 45 seconds or until you notice the texture is smooth.

Pomegranate Orange Blend

Very rich in antioxidants, this smoothie features the goodness of green tea, pomegranate, oranges, and the super food Maca. It is a true antioxidant powerhouse that is bursting with flavor.

Nutritional Info: Calories 200, Fat 0.5 g, Protein 3.9 g, Carbs 45.9 g

Servings: 2

Prep Time: 10 minutes

Ingredients:

3 oranges

1 pomegranate

1 handful parsley

1 handful carrots strips

1 musk rose (optional)

1/2 cup green tea

1 tablespoon Maca powder

6 ice cubes

Directions:

1. Wash the parsley and the carrot's stalks and remove their stems.

2. Using your juicer, juice the oranges and the pomegranate.

3. Put the resulting juice into the blender with the rest of the ingredients.

4. Blend until the mix is well combined.

5. Serve.

Full-O-Veggies

A mix of vegetables that will help you get rid of any toxins or wastes that may remain in your body after overeating. This healthy, not to mention delicious, smoothie can make for an ideal refreshing snack.

Nutritional Info: Calories 164, Fat 11.3 g, Protein 1.4g, Carbs 16.2 g

Servings: 3

Prep Time: 5 minutes

Ingredients:

1 cup natural or coconut water

1/2 avocado

2 celery stalks (chopped)

1 cup frozen strawberries

1 beet (chopped and peeled)

3 tablespoons lemon juice

1 tablespoon coconut oil

4 ice cubes

Directions:

1. Put all the ingredients into a blender.

2. Blend until the mixture is well combined and has a smooth texture.

3. Serve.

Sweet Creamy Cleanser

A rich and fresh smoothie that will fill you up with nutrients, while it helps you eliminate everything your body does not need. Enjoy this tasty fiber packed smoothie for breakfast for a week and you will feel rejuvenated.

Nutritional Info: Calories 934, Fat 77.9 g, Protein 9.9 g, Carbs 53.9 g

Servings: 1

Prep Time: 5 minutes

Ingredients:

1/2 avocado

1 frozen banana

1 cup coconut milk or pure water

1/2 cup lemon juice

5-6 fresh mint leaves

1 tablespoon vanilla extract

1 pinch of salt

Directions:

1. Put all the ingredients into a blender.

2. Blend until the mixture is well combined and has a smooth texture.

3. Serve with two mint leaves for decoration.

Blueberry Banana And Brewer's Yeast Breakfast

A fruity smoothie packed with vitamin C and antioxidants that will detoxify your body and clean it inside out. Thanks to the brewer's yeast, this smoothie is particularly advisable to cleanse the liver. You can drink this juice as replacement for breakfast for a week.

Nutritional Info: Calories 285, Fat 1.4 g, Protein 7.4 g, Carbs 68.2g

Servings: 1

Prep Time: 5 minutes

Ingredients:

1 cup frozen blueberries

1 frozen banana

1 cup grapes

1 tablespoon brewer's yeast

Ice

Directions:

1. Put all the ingredients into a blender.

2. Blend until the mixture is homogeneous and has a smooth texture.

3. You can add some water to make the smoothie lighter.

4. Serve.

Exotic Fruit And Basil Blender

A citrus smoothie featuring one of the best detoxifying fruits: pineapple. Clean your body inside out with this delicious drink and start feeling better immediately. It is advisable you drink this smoothie every day on an empty stomach for a week.

Nutritional Info: Calories 267, Fat 0.6 g, Protein 4.5 g, Carbs 67.5 g

Servings: 2

Prep Time: 5 minutes

Ingredients:

4 oranges (peeled)

1 banana

1 cup pineapple (chopped)

5 ice cubes

4 fresh basil leaves

Directions:

1. Put the oranges, the banana, and the pineapple into the blender together with the ice.

2. Blend for a minute.

3. Toss in the basil leaves and blend until they have incorporated into the mixture.

4. Serve.

Joyful Almond Banana And Pineapple

An incredibly delicious smoothie with a distinguishable nutty flavor that will fill you up with protein while it helps clean your digestive system. This smoothie will make you feel full for several hours so you can drink it early in the morning for a detoxifying effect.

Nutritional Info: Calories 351, Fat 6.1 g, Protein 6.2 g, Carbs 71.5 g

Servings: 1

Prep Time: 5 minutes

Ingredients:

8 almonds (peeled)

1 frozen banana

1 cup pineapple juice

3 tablespoons oatmeal with linseeds

Ice

Directions:

1. Put all the ingredients into a blender.

2. Blend until the mixture is homogeneous and has a smooth texture.

3. Serve.

Dinner Time Cleanser

A fruit and vegetable smoothie that is perfect for a dinner cleanse. This drink will eliminate the toxins of your body right away and at the same time, will make you feel like you have just eaten a complete meal.

Nutritional Info: Calories 134, Fat 1.3g, Protein 2.5 g, Carbs 21.3 g

Servings: 2

Prep Time: 10 minutes

Ingredients:

2 cups coconut water

1 cup frozen blueberries

1/2 cup frozen mango (chopped)

1 cup spinach leaves

1/2 cup asparagus

1 pinch cayenne pepper

1 teaspoon linseed

Ice

Directions:

1. Wash the spinach and the asparagus thoroughly.

2. Put all the ingredients into a blender.

3. Blend until the mixture is smooth and well combined.

4. Serve with some fresh mint leaves for garnishing.

Citrus And Berry Vitamin Booster

A traditional berry and citrus smoothie with a super healthy twist: the chlorella. Chlorella is packed with vitamin A, B, and C all of which will give your body a natural lift of energy and vitality.

Nutritional Info: Calories 622, Fat 28.4 g, Protein 12.5 g, Carbs 89.6g

Servings: 1

Prep Time: 5 minutes

Ingredients:

1/2 cup frozen blueberries

1/2 cup frozen raspberries

1 orange (peeled)

1 grapefruit (peeled)

1 tablespoon chlorella

1 cup coconut or almond milk

Directions:

1. Put all the ingredients into a blender.

2. Blend until the mixture is smooth and homogeneous.

3. You can add honey or stevia for extra sweetness.

4. Serve.

I Scream For Protein!

A delicious and refreshing smoothie packed with fiber, antioxidants, protein and potassium. This is truly a health powerhouse that will improve your immune system and digestive track, as well as your brain functions. It is the total package of nutrients you need.

Nutritional Info: Calories 518, Fat 22.3g, Protein 30.1 g, Carbs 51.9 g

Servings: 1

Prep Time: 5 minutes

Ingredients:

1 scoop low-fat vanilla ice cream

1 tablespoon almond butter

1 teaspoon chia seeds

1 teaspoon linseed

1 teaspoon protein powder

1 frozen banana

Ice

Directions:

1. Put all the ingredients into a blender.

2. Blend until the mixture is well combined and smooth.

3. Serve.

Spiced Spirulina Supplement

A nutritious and delightful smoothie that has high amounts of tryptophan, antioxidants, vitamin D, and protein. Thanks to the cinnamon, this drink will also lower high blood pressure, reducing stress. Add this smoothie to your daily breakfast for better results.

Nutritional Info: Calories 374, Fat 30.4 g, Protein 4.9 g, Carbs 25.3 g

Servings: 2

Prep Time: 5 minutes

Ingredients:

1 cup almond milk

1 cup coconut water

1 teaspoon spirulina

2 teaspoons chia seeds

1/4 cup frozen strawberries

1/4 cup frozen blueberries

1 tablespoon natural yogurt

A pinch of cinnamon

1 banana

Directions:

1. Put all the ingredients into a blender.

2. Blend until the mixture is well combined and smooth.

3. Serve.

The Green Goji

An appetizing smoothie with plenty of vitamins and minerals. Enjoy a cocktail of vitamin C and the benefits of the linseeds on a daily basis with this mouth-watering recipe.

Nutritional Info: Calories 313, Fat 2.8 g, Protein 8.1 g, Carbs 67.4g

Servings: 1

Prep Time: 5 minutes

Ingredients:

1 cup mixed greens (kale, lettuce, spinach)

2 frozen kiwis (peeled)

5 frozen strawberries

1 teaspoon Goji berries

1/2 cup coconut water

1 tablespoon linseed

1 teaspoon honey

Ice

Directions:

1. Put all the ingredients into the blender except for the linseeds and blend until the mix is smooth.

2. Add the linseeds and stir.

3. Serve and drink immediately.

Inflammation Buster

Both, prickly pear and aloe are known to help reduce inflammation in the walls of the stomach and intestines. All this, together with the benefits of linseeds, the chia seeds and the fruits make a delicious smoothie that will improve your digestive health.

Nutritional Info: Calories 64, Fat 0.7 g, Protein 1.4 g, Carbs 15.0 g

Servings: 4

Prep Time: 15 minutes

Ingredients:

2 grapefruits

1 cup chopped papaya

1 cup chopped pineapple

1 tablespoon linseeds

1 tablespoon chia seeds

1 leaf aloe

1/3 prickly pear

8 ice cubes

1/2 cup water

Directions:

1. Using your juicer extract the juice of the grapefruits.

2. Put the remaining ingredients into a blender together with the grapefruits' juice.

3. Blend until the mixture is well combined.

4. Serve.

Pink Is Sweet!

Let's go pink! Here comes a smoothie for Barbie doll fans!

Serves: 1-2

Ingredients:

1 cup of blueberries

1 cup of raspberries

Half avocado

1 cup of vegan milk (soy milk, rice milk, hazelnut milk—if you use soy milk, make sure it's GMO free)

Half tablespoon of soy lecithin

Some powdered nuts (I like almond powder)

Instructions:

1. Wash the blueberries and raspberries.

2. Wash and peel the avocado, remove pit, cut in half.

3. Blend all the ingredients. Serve slightly chilled with some raisins and nuts. Garnish with a slice of avocado! I recommend this smoothie for students. It's great for breakfasts or afternoon snacks. For more energy and concentration, I recommend some powdered almonds that use can squeeze in.

OPTIONAL: If your kid does not want to drink this smoothie, add some cocoa powder. Make it choco-delicious!

Anti-Cold Smoothie

This smoothie is great for winter time. You can also use it to strengthen your immune system and prevent colds and flu.

Serves: 1-2

Ingredients:

Half cup of Indian chai tea with spices (I buy it in teabags, it is a mix of black tea and spices like cardamom, clove, ginger, cinnamon, and pepper).

Half cup of vegan milk, or if you are not a vegan, goat's milk (it's mildly alkaline and much better for you than cow's milk)

1 teaspoon of cinnamon

Half clove of garlic

1 tablespoon of ginger (finely chopped)

1 banana

1 avocado

Instructions:

1. Prepare some chai tea and set aside.

2. Wash the avocado and banana. Peel and cut.

3. Blend all the ingredients and enjoy! Chai tea contains some black tea, if you are caffeine sensitive, replace with a simple yoga tea with spices (it has no theine).

As for milk—follow your own preferences. I like all kinds of vegan milk, but sometimes, I also use goat's milk. I don't drink cow's milk. Check out what works for you, and make your own choice. Cow's milk is acidic, goat's milk is slightly alkaline/neutral. In both cases, do some research, it all depends on where the milk is coming from. The same relates do cow's milk. Some brands are just full of hormones and chemicals, we don't want them in our smoothies.

Anti-Cellulite Smoothie

I recommend this smoothie as a natural energy booster, especially in the summer. If you suffer from sluggish circulation, slow bowel movement, water retention, or cellulite, try to drink it every day or at least 3 times a week.

Serves:1-2

Ingredients:
1 cup of cooled horsetail infusion (use 1-2 teabags)
1 grapefruit
1 lemon
1 cup of blueberries
1 apple
1 peach Handful of baby spinach or kale salad
Half teaspoon of spiruline powder

Instructions:
Prepare 1 cup of horsetail infusion (use 1-2 teabags) and set aside to cool down. In the meantime, wash and peel other ingredients and cut into small pieces. Mix the horsetail infusion with other ingredients; you may also add some ice cubes. Blend. Add more water or aloe vera water if needed. Add some spiruline powder, and stir energetically. Serve immediately, enjoy!

Sweet Dreams Smoothie

Can't sleep at night? Make sure you don't go to bed too hungry, but of course, don't overeat. Everyone knows this rule. How to put theory into practice? A tasty and relaxing smoothie is a great solution!

Serves:1

Ingredients:

half cup of soaked oats

1 banana

1 glass of oat milk (or other milk of your choice)

2 teaspoons of raw cocoa powder

1 teaspoon of coconut oil

Half teaspoon of cinnamon

Instructions:

Soak about half cup of oats with some warm water. Set aside. Wash, peel, and cut the banana, mix with oats, oat milk, and blend. Add 1 teaspoon of coconut oil, cocoa powder and cinnamon. Stir energetically for about a minute. Serve immediately, enjoy, relax and sleep like a baby!

I Like It Sweet!

Ok, so your kid does not like fruits/ veggies? How about trying this amazing smoothie? My tip: don't tell him /her that it contains some spinach and alga wakame...

Serves:1-2

Ingredients:
1 cup of raw almond milk or rice milk
4 teaspoons of raw cacao powder
1 tablespoon of raisins
Handful of spinach
A few raspberries
1 banana
1 teaspoon of organic honey

If your kid is active and sporty, I suggest you also add some soaked oats to give him/her more energy! Instructions: Blend and enjoy. You may want to serve it with some nuts. Superman's food!

Spanish Gazpacho Inspiration

I love Spanish gazpacho! Here's my version of "gazpaching". I have transformed the original recipe a bit to make it even healthier!

Serves:2

Ingredients:

3 cucumbers

6 tomatoes

2 red peppers

Fresh juice of 1 lemon

1 pinch of Himalaya salt (or a bit more, depends on your preferences. You may add more salt later when gazpacho is made).

2 tablespoon of olive oil

1 tablespoon of balsamic vinegar

2 pinches of black pepper (powered)

1 onion

2 carrots

1 cup of water (filtered)

2 cloves of garlic

1 cup of sweet almond milk (raw, unsweetened)

Alga wakame (cut out about 3 square centimeters, or, just cut out something that more or less resembles a size of an average cookie)

Instructions:

In a small utensil, soak wakame in some cold water (filtered). Cover, and keep for about 15 mins. In the meantime... Wash and peel all the veggies, including tomatoes (I usually soak them in some hot-boiling water so that the peel comes out) Chop the onions and garlic and the rest of the veggies. Blend all the ingredients including algae. Add more water if needed. Serve cold. Add salt, rosemary or fresh basil to taste.

MY TIP: I buy algae mix: there is some wakame, nori, agar-agar, and I just take a couple of tablespoons and soak them in water and add them to my salads, soups, and smoothies.

Spanish Salmorejo Inspiration

Here comes another recipe inspired by Spanish cuisine. Of course, I transformed it slightly. Both gazpacho and salmorejo are native to Andalucía which is south of Spain. Summers can be incredibly hot there, hence the refreshing and nourishing summer recipes like creams and soups.

Serves:2-3

Ingredients:

2 slices of toasted bread (integral, gluten-free)

2 garlic cloves

10 ripe tomatoes

100 ml of virgin olive oil

About 3-4 square centimeters of alga nori (cut it out from the leave)

Handful of spinach

1 cup of water

2 tablespoons of balsamic vinegar

Himalaya salt (1-2 pinches) and black pepper

Instructions:

1. Soak alga nori in some filtered water and leave in for 10-15 minutes.

2. In the meantime, peel the tomatoes and garlic. Wash spinach.

3. Cut the bread into small pieces.

Blend all the ingredients including alga nori. Serve cold. Season with some salt and black pepper according to your preferences. Traditionally, it is served with some hard-boiled eggs (cooled). It's up to you if you want it as a smoothie or a soup.

Super Breakfast

This is a really energizing smoothie that makes sure that you are all ready to go and smash it with your fitness goals!

Serves:1-2

Ingredients:

2 bananas

1 kiwi

1 apple

1 cup of vegan milk (I like rice milk or sweet almond milk, but can be also good quality soy milk*)

1 cup of cooked brown rice or cooked quinoa (might be a good idea to use some leftovers from your dinner)

1 teaspoon of spiruline powder

Juice of 2 grapefruits

A few leaves of kale

Instructions:

1. Wash all the fruits

2. Peel the kiwis and bananas, you can leave the apple unpeeled, it's up to you. Cut to pieces (depends on your blender preferences...)

3. Squeeze grapefruit juice.

4. Blend all the ingredients, and enjoy your workout!

Smoothie Ice-Cream

This recipe can be both a smoothie, or you can take it to a whole new level and make some delicious ice-cream! It is Paleo friendly and vegan friendly as well.

Serves:1-2

Ingredients:

2 ripe avocados

1 cup of rice milk or almond milk

A few tablespoons of raw cacao powder

2 teaspoons of organic honey (ok, you got me here, not too sure if paleos eat honey…!)

Instructions:

Wash and peel the avocados, remove the seed. Blend with other ingredients Serve cold, as a smoothie, or put in freezer for a few hours. You can add some raisins and nuts before you put it in to freeze. Enjoy your ice-cream!

Tropical Smoothie

This is a great recipe to satisfy your sweet tooth!

Serves:1-2

Ingredients:

1 mango

Half a melon

1 banana

1 kiwi

Two cups of coconut water

1 cup of filtered water

1 tablespoon of coconut oil

A few ice cubes

A few leaves of fresh mint

1 papaya

Fresh juice of 2 limes

Instructions:

Wash the fruits Peal the fruits, and remove the seeds where necessary Squeeze the limes Blend all the ingredients, and add some ice cubes if you want it super cold! Serve immediately. Garnish with some mint leaves or lime slices. So delicious! Much better option than indulging in processed sweets, right?

Herbal Smoothie

This smoothie is great for some real Paleo lovers! It is also extremely alkalizing!

Serves:1-2

Ingredients:

2 large tomatoes

1 large cucumber

Half teaspoon tablespoon cilantro

2 tablespoons parsley

1 teaspoon rosemary

1 teaspoon basil

2 cloves of garlic

1/4 teaspoon cayenne pepper

Lemon juice of 2 lemons

Optional: half cup of water

Instructions: Wash and peel the cucumber and tomatoes Squeeze some fresh lemon juice Add the herbs and blend! Serve immediately; add some ice cubes for extra refreshment. You can garnish it with some fresh mint!

Banana Spinach Berry

You can substitute a navel orange for the orange juice. You can also add a few drops of Echinacea, olive leaf extract or elderberry extract, each of which helps boost your immune system.

Serves 1.

Ingredients:

2 cups fresh spinach

¾ cup water

¾ cup orange juice

1 cup strawberries

1 cup blueberries

2 bananas

Directions:

Thoroughly wash the applicable fruits and vegetables. Blend the spinach, orange juice and water until smooth. Add everything else and blend until smooth. If you want a cold smoothie, either substitute ice for the water or freeze at least one of the other ingredients. Serve.

Tropical Green Energy

This smoothie recipe is loaded with tropical fruits and rich in antioxidants and Vitamin C. The Matcha Green Tea powder adds a subtle taste and is one of the richest sources of the antioxidant EGCG, which helps metabolism and speed up weight loss. If you are looking for a tropical treat high in vitamin C and powerful antioxidants – blend up a tropical green energy.

Ingredients:
1/2 Cup Orange Juice (Not From Concentrate)
1/2 Cup Coconut Milk (No Sugar Added)
2 tbsp Match a Green Tea Powder
1/2 Frozen Banana
1/2 Cup Frozen Mango

Directions:
Add all ingredients into a blender and whiz Enjoy!

Red Bomb Smoothie

The first summer weekend is a perfect time to try the refreshing, light and above all the special smoothie that is on the picture above. Before you start preparing salted snacks, that will in the form of salads and simple meals come on your plate, we will start with a light, nutritious and 'slender' smoothie that's very tasty.

This tasty smoothie can replace ice cream and it has only 160 calories and contains much more fiber and protein than other sweet frozen 'cousin' smoothies.

Ingredients:

1 cup of strawberries, raspberries or blueberries

Half a cup of yogurt with reduced fat content

Half a cup of juice squeezed orange or grapefruit

Preparation:

After you put all the ingredients in the blender or juicer. Mix them for about 30 seconds or 1 minute, (when you notice that all ingredients are combined into a uniform mixture). Once it's done, you can consume it immediately or cool it inside the refrigerator to make it the right summer refreshment. Knowing how to prepare a good smoothie is one of the key elements of your diet – if you want to fulfill it with healthy ingredients and fruits that are tasty, so making one every now or then can really help you lose weight.

Banana Smoothie

Settle on a sandy beach with turquoise water, choose your palm tree and enjoy the taste of the orange and banana smoothie! With the last drop, the magic will end, but, fortunately, you've prepared enough for another glass.

Ingredients:

3 oranges

1 banana

1 tablespoon of lemon juice

1 teaspoon of honey lime

Cinnamon

Preparation is rather simple, firstly squeeze the oranges and peel the banana, then with the addition of lemon juice put everything inside blender. In the end, add a teaspoon of honey, orange juice and a pinch of cinnamon.

Wild Berry Smoothie

Ingredients:

2 dl of thick yoghurt (with the smallest percentage of fat)

2 dl of milk

2 "full fists" of wild berries

2 spoons of honey

1 spoon of cinnamon

ice, if you prefer it

Preparation:

Firstly mix yogurt, milk, honey, cinnamon and butter cream with a hand blender or a regular blender. Then add frozen fruit and mix once again until you get a thick paste. Once it's prepared, pour in the glass and add one or two cubs of ice and fruit over the top – if you prefer. I add more honey to be sweeter, and I did not add the ice because the fruit was already frozen. You can also add half a ripe of a banana if you prefer it.

Apricot Smoothie

Fast, colorful and attractive – three words that describe apricot smoothie. Summer is the right time to explore different combinations of flavor and density, so choose the one you like. If you avoid milk, mix the ingredients with spring or mineral water.

Ingredients:

400 g of ripe, peeled and cleaned apricots

½ bananas (about 100 g)

2 Vanilla sugars

pinch of ground cinnamon

200 ml of natural spring water

4 tablespoons of crushed ice

Preparation:

Put apricot, banana, vanilla sugar, cinnamon and natural water in electric chopper and wait for a minute to blender do its thing. Once it's done, pour the smoothies into tall glasses, add ice (in each cup 2 tablespoons) and serve, preferably, immediately. Note. Apricots will peel more easily if you put them into boiling water.

Winter Smoothie

This is vitamin drink so tasty and full of vitamins - just what we need during these white winter days.

Ingredients:

1 orange

1 banana

2 dl of light yogurt

1 cm of fresh ginger

Preparation:

Peel orange and clean of any seeds - cut it into pieces and add pieces of bananas to the mix. Then, peeled pieces of ginger cut into smaller pieces and put in the mixer. In the end, add yoghurt. Mix everything together till you get bubbling drink, serve it and voila! During my diet I drank those 7 smoothies - because of a recommendation from my nutritionist and because my doctor told me that those are healthy - so they became my perfect replacement for high calorific food. The good thing about these smoothies is that you can drink them anytime – regardless of if you're on a diet or not because they are fresh and healthy at any time of the year.

Popeye Smoothie

This smoothie is an excellent nutritional beverage that will help you in losing weight naturally - by making your stomach full. For this smoothie, we will use almond milk (sugarless) as the main ingredient for the drink (40 calories per cup of beverage, which is considerably less than regular milk) and protein called "whey". Almond milk can be found in the local markets or you can make your own - if you find the recipe online. Mixed berries and spinach will provide you with energy and make you feel good. The overall value of this drink is only 100 calories, but it's worth it, since it's rich in proteins. Chia seeds are an excellent source of omega acids – which are also rich in dietary fiber - which will provide you with a feeling of satiety, so what are you waiting for, let's make this smoothie!

Ingredients:
1 cup of almond milk
1 cup of mixed berries (strawberries, blackberries, blueberries)
½ spinach leaves
1 cup of whey protein
45 grams of chia seed

Preparation:
Add all ingredients in a blender and mix.

Healthy Smoothie

If you are dedicated to lose weight, then this smoothie will make you rise like a phoenix. This drink is full of vitamins found in orange, pineapple and banana. Whey protein and L-Glutamine are combined together inside this smoothie to give the body a sufficient amount of amino acids and proteins. Thus prevents you from using unnecessary carbohydrates. The beverage contains less than 400 calories and has a good, refreshed taste – it's especially good after strenuous cardio exercises which I'm sure you do quite often.

Ingredients:
1 cup of orange juice
½ cup of pineapple juice
½ of banana
1 cup of whey protein
3 grams of L-glutamine

Preparation:
Add all ingredients in a blender and mix for about a minute.

Berry Flaxseed Smoothie

Flaxseeds are loaded with lignans which helps slow down tumor growth in women with breast cancer. Berry Flaxseed Smoothie is the right choice for those who want to enjoy a bit of sweetness without leaving the healthy side.

Ingredients:

½ cup mixed berries

1 banana, sliced

2 tbsp. whole flaxseed

½ cup fresh orange juice

1 cup nonfat yogurt ice

Directions:

Begin by putting the flaxseed in the blender. Blend until flaxseed is powdered. Add the orange juice, yogurt, mixed berries, and banana. Blend until thick and creamy. Sprinkle more flaxseed on top before serving.

Orange And Banana Breakfast Smoothie

Loaded with fruits, Orange and Banana Breakfast Smoothie is packed with vitamins and nutrients that you will need throughout the day.

Ingredients:

½ cup banana, sliced

¾ cup fresh orange juice

1/8 tsp. almond extract

2 tsp. brown sugar

Mint sprig

Ice

Directions:

In a blender, combine all the ingredients except the mint sprig. Blend until smooth. Add the ice cubes and blend until smooth and creamy. Garnish with mint sprig. Serve.

Very Berry Breakfast Smoothies

Start your day with this nutrient-filled smoothie. With all the berries present in this drink, this is the best antioxidant for the body.

Ingredients:

1 cup raspberries, frozen

¾ cup cherries, pitted and frozen

¾ cup almond or rice milk, unsweetened and chilled

1 ½ tbsp. honey

2 tsp. fresh ginger, finely grated

1 tsp. ground flaxseed

2 tsp. fresh lemon juice

Ice

Directions:

Combine all ingredients in a blender. Puree until smooth. Garnish by sprinkling chopped berries on top. Serve.

Apple Crumble Smoothie

Apple crumpled topped with vanilla ice cream – this smoothie will definitely leave you wanting for more!

Ingredients:

1 cup stewed apples

3 tbsp. whipped cream

1 oatmeal cookie, crumbled

¼ tsp. cinnamon

1 cup vanilla ice cream

ice

Directions:

Combine all ingredients in a blender and blend until smooth. Sprinkle with crushed oatmeal cookies on top. Serve.

Frozen Mint Lassi

This smoothie is based on fruits, spices, and flower waters, giving it an exotic but delectable taste.

Ingredients:
8 fresh mint leaves
½ cup low fat milk
2 scoops vanilla ice cream or frozen yogurt
Sugar; to taste
Mint leaves or raspberries (for garnish)
ice

Directions:
Mix low fat milk and mint leaves into your smoothie blender. Blend until mint leaves are finely chopped. Add vanilla ice cream or frozen yogurt and sugar to add taste. Pour in a glass and add extra milk if desired.

Caramel Candy Bar Smoothie

Caramel Candy Bar Smoothie is not an actual candy bar, but with all the indulgent ingredients used, it sure tastes like one – or even better!

Ingredients:

½ cup whole milk

1 scoop rich chocolate ice cream

2 scoops vanilla ice cream

1 tbsp. butterscotch sauce

2 tbsp. semisweet chocolate chips

Peanuts or almonds (for garnish)

ice

Directions:

Mix the whole milk, chocolate, butterscotch sauce, and vanilla ice cream in a blender. Pour into a glass. Add the chocolate chips. Top with the remaining vanilla ice cream and butterscotch sauce. Sprinkle with chopped peanuts or almonds. Serve.

Ginger And Pear Smoothie

This smoothie has a sweet flavor with a hint of spicy warmth due to the ginger added.

Ingredients:

1 ripe pear, chopped

1 ¼ cup ginger ice cream

2 ginger cookies, crumbled

3 tbsp. heavy whipped cream

ice

Directions:

Blend the pear, whipped cream, and ice cream in a food processor or blender. Pour into glass and top with crumbled cookies. Serve.

Pear And Cinnamon Yogurt Smoothie

Due to the clashing flavor of pear and cinnamon, this smoothie gives you a sweet and spicy taste – a mouthwatering combination that is worth a try.

Ingredients:

2 pears, peeled, cored, and chopped

¼ cup whipped cream

1 tbsp. acacia honey

1 cup full cream yogurt

1 tsp. powdered cinnamon

1 pinch nutmeg

1 pinch cinnamon sugar (for garnish)

ice

Directions:

Combine all ingredients in a blender. Pour into a glass and top off with cinnamon sugar. Serve.

Creamy Citrus Fat Burner Smoothie

This smoothie helps burn fat and improves your metabolism without losing its delicious taste.

Ingredients:
½ avocado
½ grapefruit
1 lemon, juice
1 cup dates
1 cup spinach
2 cups cooled green tea
1/3 cup nuts
1 cup coconut milk, unsweetened
2-4 drops of grapefruit therapeutic grade essential oils
ice

Directions:
Combine all ingredients except the greens and the fruits in a blender. Add the greens and blend. Add the fruits and blend until thick and smooth.

Raw Spiced Butternut Squash

This smoothie aids in weight loss, and it is very healthy and filling. Not only that, but this can also be a substitute for meals for it has oats.

Ingredients:

6 bananas, sliced

½ cup raisins

2 cups butternut squash

1 cup spinach

½ cup coconut milk, unsweetened

1 ½ cup nondairy milk

1 tsp. vanilla

¼ tsp. nutmeg

½ tsp. cinnamon

ice

Directions:

Blend in all the ingredients, adding the coconut milk and nonfat milk first. Add water if the smoothie thins out. Serve chilled.

Bananerberry Smoothie

Ingredients:

1 cup fresh strawberries

1 banana, sliced

1 cup fresh peaches

1 cup apples

1 1/2 cups vanilla ice cream

1 1/2 cups ice cubes

1/2 cup milk

Directions:

In a blender combine strawberries, banana, peaches, apples, and ice cream. Blend until smooth. Add ice, pour in milk and blend again until smooth. Serve immediately.

Hailey's Smoothie

Ingredients:

3 kiwis, peeled and chopped

2 frozen bananas, peeled and chopped

1 cup blueberries

1 cup plain yogurt

1 1/2 cups crushed ice

3 tablespoons honey

1/4 teaspoon almond extract

Directions:

In a blender, combine the kiwis, frozen bananas, blueberries, yogurt, crushed ice, honey and almond extract. Blend until smooth.

Pumpkin Pie Smoothie

Ingredients:

1 (15 ounce) can solid pack pumpkin puree

1 (12 fluid ounce) can frozen apple juice concentrate

1/8 teaspoon ground nutmeg

1 teaspoon ground cinnamon

2 1/2 cups water

Directions:

Remove pumpkin from can and freeze for 1 hour. In a blender combine partially frozen pumpkin, frozen apple juice concentrate, nutmeg and cinnamon. Blend until smooth. Continue to blend while adding water to fill the blender.

The Most Awesome Smoothie You'll Ever Make

Ingredients:

1 banana

1/2 apple

1 kiwi, peeled

1/2 cup frozen mixed berries

1 cup orange juice

1/2 cup soy milk

1/2 cup nonfat plain yogurt

1/2 cup tofu

3 tablespoons unsalted natural peanut butter

2 tablespoons aloe Vera juice

2 tablespoons flaxseed oil

1 teaspoon barley grass powder (Optional)

Directions:

In a blender, combine banana, apple, kiwi, mixed berries and orange juice. Blend until smooth. Add soy milk, yogurt, tofu, peanut butter, aloe vera juice, flaxseed oil, and barley grass powder. Blend again until well blended. Pour into glasses and serve.

Raspberry Lemon Smoothie

Ingredients:

10 ice cubes

1 1/2 cups vanilla yogurt

1 lemon, quartered and seeded

1 cup raspberries

3 tablespoons honey

Directions:

Place the ice into a blender pitcher. Add the yogurt, lemon quarters, raspberries, and honey. Cover, and blend until the mixture is smooth, or to your desired consistency. Pour into chilled glasses to serve.

Red, White, And Blue Fruit Smoothie

Ingredients:

1/2 large banana, cut into pieces and frozen

2 large fresh strawberries, rinsed and sliced

1/4 cup blueberries

1/2 cup milk

1 teaspoon vanilla extract

2 tablespoons vanilla yogurt

2 ice cubes

Directions:

Place the banana pieces, strawberries, blueberries, milk, vanilla extract, yogurt, and ice cubes in a blender. Blend until smooth.

Four-Berry Smoothies

Ingredients:

1 1/2 cups fat-free milk

1/2 cup frozen blackberries

1/2 cup frozen blueberries

1/2 cup frozen unsweetened raspberries

1/2 cup frozen unsweetened strawberries

2 tablespoons lemonade concentrate

1 tablespoon sugar

1/2 teaspoon vanilla extract

Directions:

In a blender or food processor, combine all of the ingredients. Cover and process until smooth. Pour into glasses; serve immediately.

Orange Pineapple Smoothie

Ingredients:

1 (8 ounce) can canned pineapple chunks, un-drained

1 (6 ounce) can frozen orange juice concentrate

1 cup white rum

2 tablespoons sugar

1 tablespoon lime juice

1 tray ice

4 maraschino cherries, garnish

Directions:

In a blender, combine pineapple, orange juice concentrate with juice, rum, sugar, lime juice and ice cubes. Blend until smooth. Pour into glasses, garnish with cherries, and serve.

Philadelphia 'Fruit Smoothie' No-Bake

Ingredients:

2 cups HONEY MAID Graham Cracker Crumbs

6 tablespoons butter, melted

3 tablespoons sugar

4 (8 ounce) packages PHILADELPHIA

1/3 Less Fat Cream Cheese, softened

3/4 cup sugar

1 (12 ounce) package frozen mixed berries (strawberries, raspberries, blueberries and blackberries), thawed, drained

1 (8 ounce) tub COOL WHIP LITE Whipped Topping

Directions:

Line 13x9-inch baking pan with foil, with ends of foil extending over sides of pan. Mix graham crumbs, butter and 3 Tbsp. Sugar; press onto bottom of prepared pan. Refrigerate while preparing filling. Beat cream cheese and 3/4 cup sugar in large bowl with electric mixer until well blended. Add drained berries; beat on low speed just until blended. Gently stir in whipped topping. Spoon over crust; cover. Refrigerate 4 hours or until firm. Use foil handles to remove cheesecake from pan before cutting to serve. Store leftovers in refrigerator.

Gloomy Day Smoothie

Ingredients:

1 mango - peeled, seeded, and cut into chunks

1 banana, peeled and chopped

1 cup orange juice

1 cup vanilla nonfat yogurt

Directions:

Place mango, banana, orange juice, and yogurt in a blender. Blend until smooth. Serve in clear glasses, and drink with a bendy straw!

Berry Coffee Experience

Ingredients:

1 Tablespoon Flaxseed

½ Cup Blackberries

1 Teaspoon Coffee

½ Cup Low Fat Vanilla Yogurt

½ Cup Ice Cubes

Directions:

The flaxseeds are best if they are grounded, but if not you need to blend them on high. Then you can add in the blackberries, coffee, low fat vanilla yogurt and even ice cubes. Of course, it will help you to thicken your smoothie if you freeze the blackberries. However, you will get more nutrients if you use fresh blackberries.

Why These Ingredients?

Flaxseed:

Flaxseed is a great way to stay full throughout the day, and it adds a bit of protein to your smoothies that would otherwise be lacking. Since it is a wonderful source of fiber it also keeps your digestive tract on the right track, meaning you won't hold on to unnecessary weight. Some people think it even gives you a boost of energy.

Blackberries:

Blackberries will help to naturally sweeten your smoothie, and they have weight loss benefits as well. They're also extremely high in antioxidants along with being low in calories. Blackberries also give you quick energy that can help you to work out a little earlier in the day and a little easier on top of it.

The Citrus Circus

Ingredients:

1 Cup Soy Milk

1 Teaspoon Lemon Juice

1 Teaspoon Lime Juice

1 Orange (peeled, in sections, and chilled)

1 Teaspoon Flaxseed Oil

6-7 Ice Cubes

Directions:

You can use pre-bought lime and lemon juice, but it is usually best to squeeze them fresh. Mix everything together in the blender until smooth, and then add the ice cubes until you get to the thickness of your choice. Stop adding ice cubes after you reach the desired thickness.

Why These Ingredients?

Oranges:

Oranges provide a significant amount of vitamins, which helps your body to remain healthy during the weight loss process. It also keeps your regular, which will make sure you aren't keeping on unwanted weight or bloating. Better yet, oranges has very few calories, so not many calories are added to this smoothie.

Flaxseed Oil:

Flaxseed oil is going to help provide the fiber that you need as well as start your digestive system. This will help your metabolism, and it does actually help you to stay full a little longer, which is why it has been added into this smoothie.

The Power Punch

Ingredients:

½ Cup Frozen Raspberries

1 Small Avocado (peeled and pitted)

½ Cup Oranges

2 Tablespoons Honey

½ Cup Frozen Soy Milk

Directions:

Chilling your avocado is recommended for a thicker mixture, same with your oranges. Though, it is not necessary. Just mix everything on medium until blended properly. This will usually take a few minutes since it will take time to blend the frozen fruit as well as the oranges.

Why These Ingredients?

Raspberries:

Raspberries are full of antioxidants and the vitamins that we need to stay healthy. When fighting against fat you need something that is high in fiber and not packed full of calories, and this is exactly what you get with raspberries, making it wonderful for weight loss smoothies.

Avocado:

Avocados are the right sort of fats to put into your body since they will act as an appetite suppressant, which is the main reason they were put into this weight loss smoothie.

Avocados also has a lot of fiber and nutrients that are required for healthy weight loss and general health.

Honey:

Honey provides a kick of energy and sweetness to this smoothie that was actually needed, and you will find that the energy that honey can give you is welcome. It will help to fight fatigue and help get you up and moving.

Cantaloupe Craziness

Ingredients:

8-10 Lettuce Leaves (Romaine is recommended)

2 Cups Chopped Cantaloupe

1 Cup Frozen Strawberries

5-8 Ice Cubes

Directions:

Lettuce leaves should be blended on high, as it will help to decrease the chances of stringiness. Then the chopped, and hopefully chilled, cantaloupe, strawberries, and ice cubes can be added. Blend until the thickness desired has been reached.

Why These Ingredients?

Lettuce Leaves:

Lettuce leaves are more of a filler than anything else in this weight loss smoothie recipe, but they do provide a lot of fiber. Fiber is important to healthy weight loss and control.

Cantaloupe:

Cantaloupe also provides much needed fiber for weight loss, and it is low in calories while still remaining sweet. There is no abundance in sugar, but you will find some vitamins that can also help to aid in weight loss.

Strawberries:

Strawberries are also considered to be a great way to melt away any unwanted pounds, and that is why they were added into this smoothie. Not only do they help to sweeten the smoothie, but they add much needed sugars and add fiber and potassium. Potassium is essential to workouts to avoid cramps.

Amazing Vanilla And Plum Smoothie

Ingredients:

One to two cup ice cubes

4 to 5 cups of water

5 plums

One to two vanilla bean

2 cups sugar

1/2 cup buttermilk

Preparation:

1. First cut the vanilla bean into halves and scrape the seeds.

2. Then take four cups of water in a saucepan.

3. After that combine vanilla bean extract and sugar and bring to boil.

4. Keep on stirring until the sugar is dissolved.

5. Add plums and simmer till they turn limp.

6. Withdraw the plums and deseed them.

7. Discard poaching water.

8. Now you should add plums, ice and buttermilk in a blending jar.

9. Blend till they are smoothly pureed.

10. You may now serve this smoothie at any time during the day.

Fantastic Energy Smoothie!

Ingredients:

Half to 1 of a ripe Avocado

1 cup of Vanilla flavored Yoghurt

1 Orange, peeled and sectiOned

1 cup of Strawberries (fresh or frozen)

One cup of fresh Papaya, cubed

Preparation:

1. Assemble all the Ingredients at one place.

2. Make sure you withdraw the leaves from the fruits.

3. Blend all items in a blender and blend till smooth and creamy

Serves – One to two

Time – 7 minutes

Supercool Strawberry Banana Superhuman Smoothie

Ingredients:

1 Granny Smith Apple

8 strawberries

4 mango pieces

One banana, peeled (yellow)

1 to 2 inch fresh ginger root

Preparation:

1. For this recipe you can actually use bananas that are ripe.

2. Just make sure that you drink this juice instantly after making it.

3. Don't use above-ripe mangoes though as they will make the juice taste overly tangy.

4. Blend all Ingredients in a blender or may be food processor and blend until smooth.

5. Now serve cold and topped with strawberry bits, if desired.

Strawberries Grape Banana Smoothie

Ingredients:

1/2 romaine's lettuce head

Basket of stems removed strawberries, fresh or frozen

Large handful of red grapes, seedless and stems removed

1 banana, small peeled and frozen

To create enough liquid, arrange the grapes at the bottom of a high speed blender or vitamix; and if required, add a small quantity of water to blend the other ingredients.

Directions:

Add in the fruits and green vegetables into a high speed blender or a vitamix. Just add enough water to allow the blender to bring vegetables and fruits together into a smoothie-like consistency.

Pineapple Cucumber Cleanser Smoothie

Ingredients:

1 c. of fresh or frozen pineapple

1 Celery rib

½ field of Cucumber

½ lemon, peeled

1" piece ginger

⅓ bunch parsley

1 to 2 c. of coconut water or normal water

Health Benefits:

This smoothie is very helpful of liver and kidney detoxification. Keep both of these organs supported with this smoothie as your liver has to process almost all of the substances that circulate through your body and the kidneys do a lot of work to flush out toxins from the fluids in your body.

Directions:

Place leafy greens and water into a high speed blender or a vitamix, blend until a green juice-like mixture is formed. Stop the blender and add in the remaining ingredients. Blend until creamy.

Pineapple Cucumber Cleanser Smoothie

Ingredients:

1 c. of fresh or frozen pineapple

1 Celery rib

½ field of Cucumber

½ lemon, peeled

1" piece ginger

⅓ bunch parsley

1 to 2 c. of coconut water or normal water

Health Benefits:

This smoothie is very helpful of liver and kidney detoxification. Keep both of these organs supported with this smoothie as your liver has to process almost all of the substances that circulate through your body and the kidneys do a lot of work to flush out toxins from the fluids in your body.

Directions:

Place leafy greens and water into a high speed blender or a vitamix, blend until a green juice-like mixture is formed. Stop the blender and add in the remaining ingredients. Blend until creamy.

Strawberry Banana Smoothie

Strawberry is a rich source of Boosts Memory, antioxidants. It also fights against the Cancer, relieves stress, and protects your heart. Banana helps in controlling the blood pressure, strengthens the bones, and protects your heart as well.

Ingredients:

Few strawberries, fresh or frozen

1 banana, medium

2 tsp Vanilla essence

1 tsp of Nutmeg Powder and Cinnamon Powder (optional)

¾ c. of Milk

Ice Cubes

Water and sugar, as per your desire

Directions:

Slice the bananas & the strawberries, thaw the strawberries before hand, if using frozen. Add in the banana and the strawberries in a mixer; make a thick puree of them. Add sugar and milk (not too much) and blend well. Add few ice cubes in a glass and transfer the smoothie. Before serving, top the smoothie with nutmeg powder and cinnamon powder and serve chilled.

Pineapple Cleanser Smoothie

Ingredients:

1 cup of pineapples, cut into cubes

1 part of peeled lemon

1 stalk of Celery

1/3 bundle of Parsley

½ of a Cucumber

1 piece of ginger, approximately 1 inch in length

2 cups of water (you can use coconut water if available)

Instructions:

Mix the ingredients into your juicer/blender. Blend for 20-30 seconds.

Your liver and your kidneys can greatly benefit if you drink this since the ingredients of this smoothie helps supports the processes of detoxification in these body parts.

Strawberry-Basil Green Smoothie

Ingredients:

1 peeled banana

6 medium sized strawberries

6 pieces of basil leaves

8 ounces of almond milk

2 cups of spinach

2 tablespoons of soaked (for 5 minutes) chia leaves

Instructions:

Put in the almond milk into the blender first before the other ingredients. Blend the mixture for 30 to 40 seconds until the mix becomes creamy.

If you have Vitamin deficiencies, then this smoothie is great for you. It is rich in Vitamins B1 to B6, as well as copper, potassium, phosphorous, Vitamin K and magnesium. It has 11 grams of fiber, which aids in proper digestion.

Super Detox Green Cleansing Smoothie

Ingredients:

1 piece of pear, small and cut into cubes

1 piece of banana, chopped

1 cup of romaine leaves, torn

1 cup of spinach leaves (you can also use kale leaves)

½ cup of chopped cucumbers

½ cup of chopped celery

½ piece of lemon, with the juice extracted

1 cup of water (you can also use coconut water if available)

1 tablespoon of mint, fresh

1 tablespoon of parsley, fresh

1 slice of peeled ginger, ¼ inch in size

½ tablespoon of chia seeds

Optional: 1 pinch of cinnamon, 1 pinch of cayenne and 1 pinch of turmeric

Instructions:

Mix all the ingredients in a blender until a smooth texture is achieved. Sweeten as necessary.

This smoothie recipe is a great recipe that you can try because of the benefits that ou can reap out of it. It has no cholesterol, low in sodium, high in potassium and high in Vitamin A, B6 and C. It is also high in dietary fiber and manganese.

The Super Green Smoothie

Ingredients:

1 ¼ cup of frozen mango, cut into cubes

1 ¼ cup of Lacinato kale leaves, chopped

¼ cup of parsley, chopped

¼ cup of mint, chopped

1 cup of fresh orange juice

2 stalks of fresh celery, chopped

Instructions:

Mix all of the ingredients in a blender and puree until the texture becomes smooth and creamy.

This smoothie recipe includes several ingredients that have diuretic properties that can help in eliminating toxins out of our bodies.

The Breakfast Blend

Ingredients:

2 cups of spinach

1 ½ cups of blueberries

¼ cup of superfood greens

2 cups of almond milk, unsweetened

1 piece of banana

1 teaspoon of spirulina Ice cubes

Instructions:

Blend all of the ingredients until it becomes creamy, frothy and smooth.

This smoothie recipe is a great replacement for a breakfast meal. It can help you feel energized and alert.

The Super Hemp

Ingredients:

½ piece of banana, sliced

2 cups of blueberries

1 cup of coconut almond milk

1 tablespoon of superfood greens

1 cup of spinach

1 tablespoon of spirulina

2 tablespoons of hemp protein powder

Instructions:

Blend all of these fruits and vegetables in a blender and add a teaspoon of hempseed oil if you necessary.

This smoothie blend is a great thing to enjoy at lunch. You can replace your unhealthy lunch meal with this and acquire essential nutrients and minerals without feeling guilty.

Alkalinity Bliss

Ingredients:

¼ piece of avocado, chopped

1 teaspoon of chia seeds

1 cup of spinach ½ piece of pear, chopped

1 scoop of hemp protein powder

¼ cup of coconut water

1 cup of almond milk Water

Instructions:

Put all of the ingredients into the blender and blend for 30 to 35 seconds.

This recipe features chia seeds which contains 2 grams of dietary fiber. If that alone already makes it a healthy substitute to sugar filled drinks, then tune out for more because it also comes with other fruits and vegetables that surely have healthy benefits for the body.

The Ultimate Green Smoothie Detox

Ingredients:

½ piece of peeled lime

1 piece of peeled orange

2 cups of chopped kale or dandelion greens

1 piece of medium sized banana, peeled and sliced

1 tablespoon of soaked (for 5 minutes) chia seeds

1 small piece of ginger, grated

8 ounces of water (you can also use homemade almond milk if available)

Instructions:

Except for the greens, blend all of the ingredients and push the "pulse" button for a couple of times. Set the blender on "high" and add the greens. Blend for 30 seconds or so.

This smoothie recipe is so great that it contains 9 grams of protein, 64 grams of carbohydrates, 321 calories and 25% of calcium. And oh, it also contains 4.2 grams of iron. Simply amazing!

Cilantro Detox Smoothie

Ingredients:

2 stalks of celery

1/3 bundle of fresh cilantro

½ cup of fresh pineapples, chopped into cubes

1 cup of green lettuce leaves

1 piece of ginger root, 1 inch in size

2 cups of coconut water

Instructions:

Blend all of the ingredients well in a blender. Puree until the texture becomes smooth.

This recipe will help eliminate heavy metals inside your body since one of its ingredients is cilantro. Since it also features the popular pineapple, it is also good for digestion.

Green And Clean Smoothie

Ingredients:

1 stalk of celery

2 sprigs of fresh mint

½ piece of avocado, sliced

¼ piece of cucumber, sliced

1 piece of kiwi

½ fistful of spinach

½ piece of pineapple

1 cup of purified water

A little hint of lemon juice

Instructions:

Simply blend all of the ingredients using a blender and wait for the texture of the mixture to turn smooth.

This smoothie recipe features everything green. You can benefit from all the fiber and nutrients, not to mention that mineral and the vitamins, which the ingredients of this delicious and healthy smoothies have.

Classic Green Juice

Ingredients:

1 small Granny Smith apple

¼ English cucumber or 1 small Israeli cucumber

1 small bunch of kale

1 handful green grapes

This juice is full of iron and vitamin K – just the thing for drinking before your menstrual cycle.

Dairy Berry Green Smoothie

Ingredients:

½ cup spinach

½ cup sliced bananas

½ cup blueberries

½ cup non- dairy milk

½ cup oats

1 tablespoon sunflower seeds

½ cup ice cubes

½ cup water

Instructions:

Put ice cubes, water, spinach and oats in a blender. Blend on high speed until mixed. Add milk blueberries, bananas and sunflower seeds. Blend until smooth. Pour into a tall glass and serve.

Ready for something a little outside the box? This mouthwatering smoothie is a combination of tart blueberries, sweet banana, and an effervescent twist. Sunflower seeds just a little something that will leave you thinking and wanting more! Try sharing this daring drink and see if your friends and family can guess the secret ingredient.

Grape Celery Power Smoothie

Ingredients:

1 cup black grapes.

1 large stalk of celery

½ cup instant oats

1 tablespoon pumpkin seeds

½ cup oat milk

½ cup coconut water

½ cup ice cubes

Instructions:

Cut celery into 2-inch strips so it becomes easier to process. Put celery, oats, ice cubes and water in a blender and whiz on high speed until smooth. Add black grapes, pumpkin seed and milk blend until smooth. Pour into a glass and drink fresh.

Believe it or not, coconut water has been administered to dehydrated patients via IV straight into their veins. This is because it is perfectly balanced to restore the body's fluids and is full of electrolytes. After a long day at work or a good workout, it's not uncommon to feel dehydrated. This soothing smoothie is the perfect way to replenish your body's water balance while indulging in a delicious treat. This smoothie also helps you with your joint pains, lung infections and asthma.

Vanilla Coconut Green Smoothie

Ingredients:

1 cup kale leaves

½ cup Oats

½ teaspoon vanilla extract

A pinch of salt

¼ cup unsweetened coconut milk

½ cup ice cubes

Instructions:

Blend kale leaves and water first. When smooth, add oats, Vanilla extract, salt, coconut milk and ice cubes and blend until fully mixed. Pour into a glass and serve.

When you think of a powerhouse of nutrition, dark leafy greens always come to mind. They are a great source of vitamins like B, K, C, and E along with many essential minerals. This smoothie is a great one for those of you who are trying to become more accustomed to the flavor of greens. That's because I paired them up with tangy green and sweet vanilla for a smoothie that is green, but with a hint of sweetness.

Lemon Forest Green Smoothie

Ingredients:

½ cup pineapple

¼ cup cauliflower florets

½ cup pink grapefruit

½ tablespoon linseeds

1 tablespoon lemon zest

½ tablespoon almond nuts

2 tablespoon dried pitted dates (pre-soaked for a smoother blend)

1/4 cup dried apricots

½ cup non- dairy milk

Instructions:

Put water, milk, broccoli, Pineapple, cauliflower and grapefruit in a blender. Whiz until, mixed thoroughly. Add linseeds, almonds, dates and apricots. Blend until smooth. Pour into a tall glass and enjoy.

Dreamy and creamy, this smoothie is like a melted Popsicle in a cup. And even though it's green, you'd never guess by its bright and fresh flavor that cauliflower florets have worked its way into the mix. Don't let the sweet, light flavor fool you either. This smoothie is packed with iron, protein, and fiber which make for a substantial drink.

Yogurt Peach Green Smoothie

Ingredients:

1 cup romaine lettuce

3 small whole peaches

1 tablespoon sesame seeds

¼ cup dried apricots(pre-soaked for a smoother blend)

½ cup non – dairy milk

½ cup non-dairy yogurt

½ cup ice cubes

Instructions:

Blend in romaine lettuce, milk and yogurt until smooth. Add all remaining ingredients and process in the blender until thoroughly, mixed. Pour into a glass and drink immediately.

For me, the heavy green flavor of dark leafy vegetables has been an acquired taste. That doesn't apply to this smoothie. Because of the addition of fresh flavors like dill, romaine lettuce, and citrus this smoothie is light and refreshing. It's a tasty combination that, if you are not a greens person, you will be glad you tried.

Green Hurricane Delta Detox Smoothie

Ingredients:

½ cup spinach

½ kale leaves

¼ romaine lettuce

4 broccoli heads

Medium stalk of celery

¼ cup parsley leaves

¼ cup Brussels sprouts

5 mint leaves

3 medium lemon

Pinch of sea salt

1 cup ice cubes

Instructions:

First peel lemon and square them. Put rest of the ingredient in the blender. Whiz until smooth Pour into glass and drink fresh.

This smoothie is dedicated to all of the die-hard green smoothie addicts out there. This is the most hard core leafy green smoothie in this book. Please don't let that scare you off, though. The fresh lime lightens up the flavor quite a bit. There's even a bit of neutral zucchini thrown in the mix for a balanced, yet unmistakably green, drink.

Minty Green Smoothie

Ingredients:

1 cup chopped spinach leaves

10 pieces mint leaves

2 whole pitted dates

2 tablespoons raw cashew butter

1 ½ cups distilled water

Instructions:

Put all ingredients in a blender. Whiz on high speed until smooth. Pour into glasses and serve immediately.

Variation: Substitute pitted dates with 1 tablespoon of raw coconut nectar or raw agave nectar Add 1 cup of ice cubes for a cold treat.

Mint not only triggers a feeling of satiety (it makes you feel full!) but also helps flush out toxins from the digestive tract. It also aids in proper digestion by soothing the intestines and loosening intestinal muscles, thus relieving cramps and other symptoms of disturbed stomach.

Tropical Blast Green Smoothie

Ingredients:

1 cup of pineapple

1 cup of mango

1 cup of banana

¾ cup of spinach

2 cups of fresh coconut water, almond milk, or clean, filtered water

6 ice cubes (optional)

Instructions:

Make sure to thoroughly rinse and clean the spinach in clean water. Dice the pineapple, mango and banana to measure one cup. Add all ingredients to your blender (add spinach last). Blend for 30 seconds to 1 minute, depending on speed setting. Let the ingredients blend until creamy.

Mangoes are highly effective in soothing the GI tract and optimizing your digestion. Furthermore, the pretty fruits are rich in vitamin C, providing an essential immune system boost. Pineapples contribute to weight loss because they have a very high water and fiber content. High water/fiber content foods make you feel satisfied; so another snack is not necessary. Furthermore, pineapples have been shown to naturally curb your appetite.

Savory & Spicy Green Smoothie

Ingredients:

1 whole avocado

1 lemon

1 orange beet (small)

1 cucumber (small)

5 stalks of collards greens

2 drops of vanilla extract

1 inch-thick piece of ginger

½ of a jalapeno pepper

Instructions:

Remove the seeds and skin from the lemon, and add them to the blender. Cut cucumber, orange beet, and collard greens into smaller chunks, then add the collard greens to the blender last. Place the ginger, avocado, jalapeno (with seeds) and clean water in the blender's pitcher last. Blend until the green smoothie reaches your desired consistency. *Wash the collards, cucumber, and jalapeno thoroughly before adding to blender.

Jalapeno peppers lend an essential nutritional punch to your green smoothie. One of the jalapeno pepper's key nutrients is capsaicin; it revs your metabolism and boosts your immune system. It further increases your blood flow, weight loss capabilities, and boosts your energy. Ginger is excellent to ward off cancers and interior muscle soreness. It further works to alleviate nausea. This smoothie also serves as a great meal replacement for breakfast; it's rich and filling and will keep you full and energized throughout a busy morning. It will also decrease your likelihood of snacking on other processed foods!

Electrolyte Balancer Green Smoothie

Ingredients:

2 cups of fresh pineapple

2 fresh celery ribs, chopped

1 cup of spinach

1 lime (without skin and seeds)

2 cups of coconut milk

Instructions:

Before adding the celery and spinach to the blender, first thoroughly soak & rinse them with water. Then in the blender's pitcher, add the chopped pineapple chunks, celery, lime, coconut milk and spinach; allow all of the fresh ingredients to blend until they reach a creamy, smooth texture.

When you want to enhance your electrolyte and hormonal balance, you must look to the beneficial effects of both coconut milk and celery. Furthermore, when you add pineapple, this smoothie fights back against certain strains of bacteria and infections. It further acts as nourishment for both your hair and skin.

Orange-Banana Green Smoothie

Ingredients:

1 cup spinach

1 large banana

2 celery ribs

2 oranges (peeled)

1 coconut water or filtered water

Instructions:

Allow the spinach and celery to soak in water to remove any impurities. Afterwards, add oranges, celery, banana, and coconut water to the blender. Make sure to add the spinach last, and allow the mix to blend until it is creamy enough for your preference.

If you're opting for orange's pulsing nutrients, it's best to look to the natural variety for assistance. Store-bought orange juice has been sitting on the shelves for days and days. Many orange juice products consist of only water and synthetic orange flavoring (with no nutrition at all!). When you utilize freshly blended or juiced oranges, you are getting a higher value of vitamin A & C, both of which are crucial for your body to fend off toxins, pathogens, and bacteria. Remember: when it comes to fruits and vegetables, fresh is always best!

Sweet Kiwi Green Smoothie

Ingredients:

2 leaves kale (without stems)

1 medium cucumber (peeled)

2 kiwis (without skin)

2 Medjool dates (pitted)

1 cup of coconut water (or clean water)

Instructions:

First wash the kale and cucumber. Dice both and add the cucumber to the blender, along with the kiwis, dates and coconut water. Add the kale last while blending. Allow the mixture of fruits and vegetables to blend until they reach your desired consistency.

The vibrant green kiwis contain high levels of omega 3 fatty acids, something usually found in nuts and very rarely in fruits. Remember that your brain requires a balance in the brain of omega-3 fatty acids because they create better cell-to-cell communication, fueling necessary hormonal balances. Furthermore, kiwis are a great source of potassium and vitamin C. Recent research states that kiwis are especially effective in the prevention of cellular oxidation. Remember that cellular oxidation is the event in which free radicals kill cells by removing one of their electrons and forcing protein and DNA death. This hinders the cell's ability to communicate with surrounding cells and eventually kills it. Cucumbers contain silica, a trace mineral that increases the body's ability to heal skin wounds. This mineral can also assist with strengthening the skin's connective tissues.

Blueberry Smoothie

Ingredients:

1 c skim milk

1 c frozen unsweetened blueberries

Instructions:

1. Combine milk and blueberries in blender, and blend for 1 minute.
2. Transfer to glass, and stir in flaxseed oil.
3. Drink fresh.

Blueberries considered a "superfood", are low in calories but high in nutrients and super healthy. They contain Fiber, Vitamin C, Vitamin K and Manganese. Blueberries reduce DNA damage, which may help protect against ageing and cancer, lower blood pressure, protect LDL lipoproteins (the "bad" cholesterol) from oxidative damage, prevent heart disease, improve brain function and memory, has anti-diabetic effects, prevents urinary tract infections, help reduce muscle damage after intensive exercise.

Apple Low Carb Smoothie

Ingredients:

2 large green apples cored

1 frozen banana

1 cup ice

1 cup unsweetened almond milk

1/ 2 cup Greek yogurt

Instructions:

1. Add all ingredients to a blender.

2. Pulse until combined and smooth.

3. Taste and add sweetener if desired, pulsing to combine.

4. Serve immediately.

5. Sprinkle the top of each smoothie with a pinch of cinnamon.

6. Drink fresh.

"An apple a day keeps the doctor away". Apples are known to improve neurological health, prevent dementia, reduce the risk of stroke, reduce the risk of diabetes, help prevent breast cancer, prevent bad cholesterol in blood from rising, protect the body from the free radicals.

Detox Green Smoothie

Ingredients:

1 stalk kale, stem removed

1 cup baby spinach/ greens

1/ 2 lemon, seeds removed, skin on

1/ 2 inch piece of peeled ginger

3 inch piece of peeled cucumber

Instructions:

1. Combine all ingredients in a blender and blend until smooth.

2. Drink fresh.

Kale is high in iron, in Vitamin K, filled with powerful antioxidants, has anti-inflammatory properties and cardiovascular support substances, high in Vitamin A, Vitamin C, calcium and is a great detox food, keeping the liver healthy.

Pineapple Spinach Detox Smoothie

Ingredients:

3/ 4 cup pineapple juice

1/ 2 cup fresh spinach leaves

1/ 4 pear, chopped

1/ 4 green apple, chopped

1/ 4 avocado, chopped

Instructions:

1. Blend pineapple juice, spinach, pear, apple, avocado, and broccoli together in a blender until smooth.

2. Drink fresh.

Pineapples improves respiratory health, improves digestion, strengthens bones, reduces inflammation, prevents cancer, increases heart health, reduces infections and parasites, strengthens the immune system, and increases circulation.

Pear Avocado Smoothie

Ingredients:

½ pear

¼ avocado

½ cucumber

½ lemon

handful of cilantro

1 cup kale (packed)

½ inch ginger

½ cup coconut water

1 scoop protein powder (hemp, pumpkin or pea works great!)

Water

Instructions:

1. Blend all ingredients until smooth.
2. Drink fresh.

The health benefits of avocado include weight management, protection against cardiovascular diseases, diabetes, osteoarthritis and enhancing the absorption of nutrients. It also reduces the risk of cancer, liver damage and Vitamin K deficiency-related bleeding. Keeps eyes healthy and protects the skin from aging and from harmful effects of UV rays. It also helps in maintaining normal blood sugar levels and has antioxidant properties, boosts cognitive abilities, and build stronger bones!

Papaya Smoothie

Ingredients:

1 cup papaya

1 cup coconut kefir, coconut yogurt or coconut milk

juice from ½ lime

1 tbsp. raw honey

Instructions:

1. Blend all ingredients until smooth.

2. Drink fresh.

Papaya is rich in fiber, improves digestion, rich in Vitamin C and antioxidants, lowers cholesterol, boosts immunity, good for diabetics, great for the eyes, protects against arthritis, prevents signs of ageing and cancer and helps reduce stress.

Peaches And Pineapples Green Smoothie

Ingredients:

1 cup unsweetened almond milk

1/ 2 cup frozen pineapple

2 cups kale

1/ 2 banana

1 cup frozen peaches

Instructions:

Prepare all the ingredients and put them in a blender. Pulse on medium speed.Process until smooth. When the mixture becomes smooth and creamy, transfer it into your glass and serve.

Power up your day with powerful combinations of fruits such as peaches, pineapples, bananas, and spinach. Peaches is a good source of antioxidants with a long list of benefits including its anti-inflammatory, anti-cancer, and anti-aging effects. Banana, on the other hand, is rich in potassium. You also have pineapples with bromelain, which aids in inflammation and is good for the heart. Top all these with spinach and you are in for some flavorful and nutritious smoothie.

www.ingramcontent.com/pod-product-compliance
Lightning Source LLC
Chambersburg PA
CBHW071400280526
45787CB00001B/398